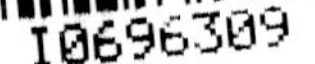

ESSENTIAL SUPPLEMENTS FOR ENHANCING FERTILITY

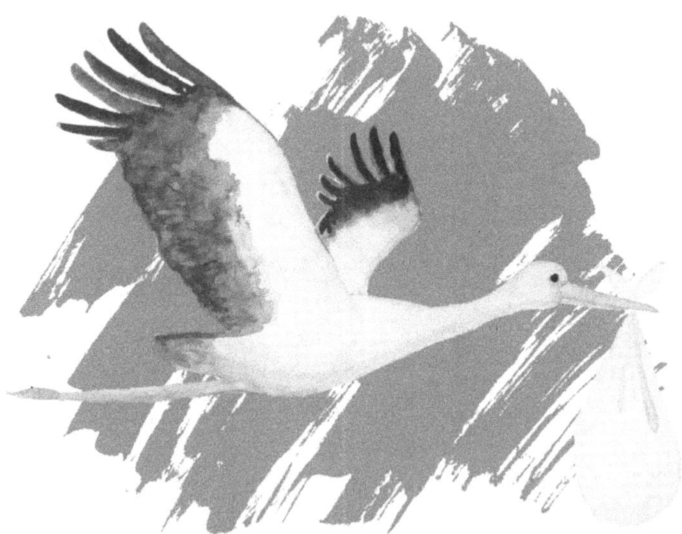

Aurora Brooks

xspurts.com

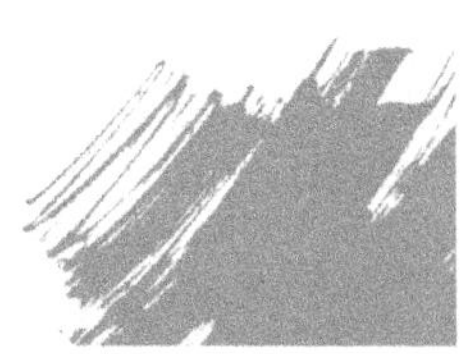

Free Book Offer:
<u>Get How to be a Super Mom For Free</u>

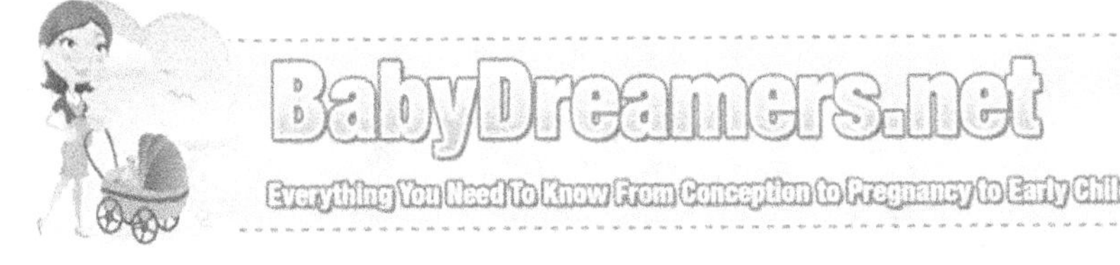

A Short Read is a type of book that is designed to be read in one quick sitting.

These no fluff books are perfect for people who want an overview about a subject in a short period of time.

Table of Contents

GARLIC

VITAMIN K

RESVERATROL

NETTLE LEAF

ANTIOXIDANT BLEND

ASHWAGANDHA

CHROMIUM

FREQUENTLY ASKED QUESTIONS

Have Questions / Comments?

Get How To Be A Super Mom 100% FREE

Essential Supplements for Enhancing Fertility

When it comes to enhancing fertility and increasing the chances of conception, incorporating essential supplements into your daily routine can make a significant difference. These supplements are packed with nutrients that support reproductive health and address any deficiencies that may be hindering fertility.

Exploring the benefits of various supplements can help you understand how they can improve fertility and increase your chances of conceiving. From supporting healthy ovulation and sperm production to enhancing egg quality and hormone regulation, these supplements offer a holistic approach to fertility enhancement.

Let's delve into the world of essential supplements for enhancing fertility and discover how they can positively impact your reproductive health.

Folic Acid

Folic Acid

Folic acid, also known as folate or vitamin B9, plays a crucial role in promoting fertility and ensuring a healthy pregnancy. It is particularly important for women who are trying to conceive as it helps in preventing birth defects and supporting healthy ovulation. Folic acid is essential for the development of the neural tube in the early stages of pregnancy, which eventually forms the baby's brain and spinal cord. Adequate intake of folic acid before and during pregnancy can significantly reduce the risk of neural tube defects such as spina bifida.

In addition to its role in preventing birth defects, folic acid also supports healthy ovulation in women and sperm production in men. It aids in the production of DNA and RNA, the building blocks of genetic material, which are crucial for the development of healthy eggs and sperm. Folic acid also plays a role in regulating hormone levels and promoting overall reproductive health.

It is recommended that women of childbearing age consume 400-800 micrograms of folic acid daily, either through a balanced diet or supplements. Good dietary sources of folic acid include leafy green vegetables, citrus fruits, beans, and fortified cereals. However, it can be challenging to obtain sufficient amounts of folic acid through diet alone, especially for women who are planning to conceive. Therefore, taking a folic acid supplement is highly recommended to ensure optimal levels for fertility and pregnancy.

Iron

Iron plays a crucial role in fertility for both men and women. Iron deficiency can have a significant impact on reproductive health and increase the risk of infertility. In women, iron deficiency can lead to irregular menstrual cycles, making it difficult to predict ovulation and conceive. It can also affect the quality of eggs produced and hinder their ability to be fertilized.

For men, iron deficiency can impair sperm production and motility, reducing the chances of successful fertilization. Low iron levels can also affect the quality and quantity of sperm, making it more challenging for couples to conceive.

Supplementing with iron is essential to address iron deficiency and improve fertility outcomes. Iron supplements can help replenish iron stores in the body and support healthy reproductive function. It is important to consult with a healthcare professional to determine the appropriate dosage and duration of iron supplementation.

In addition to iron supplements, it is also important to include iron-rich foods in the diet. Good sources of iron include lean meats, poultry, fish, beans, lentils, spinach, and fortified cereals. Combining iron-rich foods with foods high in vitamin C can enhance iron absorption.

Ensuring adequate iron levels can optimize fertility for both men and women, increasing the chances of conception and a healthy pregnancy. By addressing iron deficiency through supplementation and a balanced diet, couples can take proactive steps towards enhancing their fertility.

Vitamin D

Vitamin D plays a crucial role in fertility and reproductive health. A deficiency in vitamin D can have a significant impact on a couple's ability to conceive. Research has shown that low levels of vitamin D in both men and women can lead to decreased fertility and an increased risk of infertility.

One of the main benefits of vitamin D supplementation is its ability to improve reproductive health. Vitamin D helps regulate hormone levels, including those involved in the menstrual cycle and sperm production. It also supports the development and maturation of eggs and sperm, increasing the chances of successful fertilization.

Furthermore, vitamin D deficiency has been linked to an increased risk of conditions that can negatively affect fertility, such as polycystic ovary syndrome (PCOS) and endometriosis. By ensuring adequate levels of vitamin D through supplementation, couples can potentially improve their chances of conception and reduce the risk of these reproductive disorders.

In addition to its direct impact on fertility, vitamin D is also essential for overall reproductive health. It plays a role in maintaining a healthy immune system, reducing inflammation, and supporting the development of a healthy pregnancy. Adequate levels of vitamin D have been associated with a lower risk of pregnancy complications, such as gestational diabetes and preterm birth.

To ensure optimal fertility and reproductive health, it is recommended to have your vitamin D levels checked and consider supplementation if deficiency is detected. The dosage and duration of supplementation should be determined by a healthcare professional based on individual needs and circumstances.

Coenzyme Q10

Coenzyme Q10, also known as CoQ10, is a powerful antioxidant that plays a crucial role in enhancing fertility for both men and women. This essential nutrient is naturally produced by the body and is found in every cell, especially in the mitochondria, where it helps convert food into energy.

When it comes to fertility, CoQ10 has been found to have significant benefits. For women, it can enhance egg quality, which is essential for successful conception and healthy pregnancies. As women age, the quality of their eggs naturally declines, making it more challenging to conceive. CoQ10 supplementation can help counteract this decline by improving egg health and increasing the chances of successful fertilization.

For men, CoQ10 can improve sperm motility, which refers to the ability of sperm to move efficiently towards the egg. Motility is a crucial factor in male fertility, as it determines the sperm's ability to reach and penetrate the egg for fertilization. By enhancing sperm motility, CoQ10 can increase the chances of successful conception for couples trying to conceive.

Furthermore, CoQ10 has been found to have potential benefits for couples undergoing assisted reproductive technologies, such as in vitro fertilization (IVF). Studies have shown that CoQ10 supplementation can improve the success rates of IVF by increasing the number of high-quality embryos and improving overall reproductive outcomes.

To incorporate CoQ10 into your fertility-enhancing regimen, it is recommended to take a daily supplement. The dosage may vary depending on individual needs, so it is best to consult with a healthcare professional for personalized guidance. Additionally, CoQ10-rich foods include organ meats, fatty fish, and whole grains, which can be incorporated into a balanced diet to support fertility.

Vitamin C

Vitamin C is a powerful antioxidant that plays a crucial role in maintaining reproductive health for both men and women. As an antioxidant, vitamin C helps to protect the reproductive cells from oxidative damage caused by free radicals. This protection is especially important for sperm, as oxidative stress can lead to DNA damage and decreased sperm quality.

For men, vitamin C has been shown to improve sperm quality by increasing sperm count, motility, and morphology. It also helps to prevent sperm clumping, which can hinder fertility. Additionally, vitamin C has been found to reduce the risk of sperm DNA damage, which is associated with lower fertility rates.

In women, vitamin C has positive effects on reproductive health as well. It helps to support the production of healthy cervical mucus, which is essential for sperm survival and transport. Adequate levels of vitamin C also promote the development of healthy eggs and can improve the chances of successful fertilization.

It's important to note that vitamin C is a water-soluble vitamin, which means it is not stored in the body and needs to be replenished regularly. Including vitamin C-rich foods in your diet, such as citrus fruits, berries, and leafy greens, can help ensure you're getting an adequate intake. However, if you're trying to conceive or have specific fertility concerns, you may consider supplementing with vitamin C to ensure optimal levels.

In conclusion, vitamin C is a valuable nutrient for enhancing sperm quality and supporting female reproductive health. Its antioxidant properties help to protect reproductive cells from oxidative damage, improving fertility outcomes for both men and women. Whether through diet or supplementation, ensuring an adequate intake of vitamin C is an important step towards optimizing fertility.

Zinc

Zinc plays a crucial role in fertility, as it is involved in various processes that are essential for reproductive health. One of the key functions of zinc is its role in hormone regulation. Zinc helps in the production and release of hormones that are necessary for the menstrual cycle and ovulation in women. In men, zinc is important for the production of testosterone, which is vital for sperm production and maturation.

In addition to hormone regulation, zinc also plays a role in sperm production. It is a key component of the genetic material in sperm and is necessary for the development of healthy sperm. Zinc deficiency can lead to decreased sperm count, poor sperm quality, and impaired fertility in men.

To ensure adequate zinc levels for optimal fertility, it is important to include zinc-rich foods in your diet or consider zinc supplementation. Foods rich in zinc include oysters, beef, lamb, pumpkin seeds, and spinach. However, it is important to note that excessive zinc intake can also have negative effects on fertility, so it is best to consult with a healthcare professional for guidance on the appropriate dosage.

In conclusion, zinc plays a vital role in fertility by regulating hormones and supporting sperm production. Ensuring adequate zinc levels through a balanced diet or supplementation can help enhance fertility and increase the chances of conception.

Omega-3 Fatty Acids

Omega-3 fatty acids are essential nutrients that play a crucial role in improving fertility, reducing inflammation, and supporting overall reproductive health. These healthy fats are found in abundance in fatty fish, such as salmon, mackerel, and sardines, as well as in flaxseeds, chia seeds, and walnuts.

One of the key benefits of omega-3 fatty acids is their ability to enhance fertility. Research suggests that these fats can improve egg quality in women and increase sperm count and motility in men. By incorporating omega-3-rich foods or supplements into your diet, you can optimize your reproductive health and increase your chances of conceiving.

In addition to their fertility-enhancing properties, omega-3 fatty acids also have powerful anti-inflammatory effects. Inflammation in the body can disrupt hormone balance and impair reproductive function. By reducing inflammation, omega-3s can help create a more favorable environment for conception and pregnancy.

Furthermore, omega-3 fatty acids support reproductive health by promoting proper hormone production and function. These fats are involved in the synthesis of hormones that regulate the menstrual cycle and support healthy ovulation. By ensuring an adequate intake of omega-3s, you can help maintain hormonal balance and optimize your reproductive system.

To incorporate omega-3 fatty acids into your diet, consider adding fatty fish, flaxseeds, chia seeds, and walnuts to your meals. If you're unable to consume enough of these foods, omega-3 supplements are also available. However, it's important to consult with a healthcare professional before starting any new supplements to ensure they are safe and appropriate for your individual needs.

Probiotics

Probiotics:

The impact of gut health on fertility is often overlooked, but it plays a crucial role in reproductive health for both men and women. The gut microbiome, which consists of trillions of bacteria and other microorganisms, influences various aspects of our overall health, including fertility.

Probiotics, which are beneficial bacteria, can be taken as supplements to support and improve gut health. These supplements help maintain a healthy balance of bacteria in the gut, which in turn can have positive effects on fertility.

For women, a healthy gut microbiome is essential for proper hormone regulation and menstrual cycle regularity. Imbalances in gut bacteria can lead to hormonal disruptions, irregular periods, and even conditions like polycystic ovary syndrome (PCOS). By taking probiotics, women can support a healthy gut microbiome and potentially improve their fertility.

For men, gut health is also important for reproductive function. Studies have shown that imbalances in gut bacteria can negatively impact sperm quality and motility. By taking probiotics, men can help optimize their gut health and potentially enhance their fertility.

Probiotics can be particularly beneficial for couples undergoing fertility treatments, such as in vitro fertilization (IVF). These treatments can disrupt the natural balance of gut bacteria, and taking probiotics can help restore that balance and support the success of the treatments.

It's important to note that not all probiotics are the same, and it's essential to choose a high-quality supplement that contains strains of bacteria known to have positive effects on fertility. Consulting with a healthcare professional or fertility specialist can help determine the most suitable probiotic supplement for individual needs.

In addition to supplements, incorporating probiotic-rich foods into the diet can also support gut health. Foods like yogurt, kefir, sauerkraut, and kimchi are rich in beneficial bacteria and can help maintain a healthy gut microbiome.

In summary, the impact of gut health on fertility should not be underestimated. Probiotic supplementation can help support a healthy gut microbiome, regulate hormones, and improve reproductive function for both men and women. Whether trying to conceive naturally or undergoing fertility treatments, incorporating probiotics into the daily routine can be a beneficial step towards enhancing fertility.

Calcium

Calcium:

Calcium plays a vital role in reproductive health, particularly in the proper functioning of hormones and the fertilization of eggs. This essential mineral is not only important for building strong bones and teeth but also for supporting various physiological processes in the body.

When it comes to fertility, calcium is crucial for the regulation of hormones involved in the menstrual cycle and ovulation. It helps maintain the balance of estrogen and progesterone, which are essential for the release of mature eggs and the preparation of the uterus for implantation. Calcium also aids in the contraction and relaxation of the uterine muscles during the menstrual cycle and pregnancy.

In addition to its role in hormone function, calcium is essential for the fertilization of eggs. It is involved in the activation of sperm cells, allowing them to penetrate and fertilize the egg. Calcium also plays a crucial role in the development of the fertilized egg, supporting its growth and division.

Ensuring an adequate intake of calcium is essential for both men and women who are trying to conceive. While dairy products are often considered the primary source of calcium, there are also other options available, such as fortified plant-based milk, leafy greens, tofu, and almonds. It is important to note that calcium absorption is enhanced when consumed with vitamin D, so it is beneficial to include sources of both nutrients in the diet.

Overall, calcium plays a significant role in reproductive health by supporting proper hormone function and facilitating egg fertilization. Including calcium-rich foods in your diet can help optimize fertility and increase the chances of conception.

Vitamin E

Vitamin E is a powerful antioxidant that plays a crucial role in improving fertility and reproductive outcomes. As an antioxidant, it helps protect the reproductive cells from oxidative damage caused by free radicals, which can negatively impact fertility. By neutralizing these harmful molecules, vitamin E helps maintain the integrity of the reproductive cells and supports healthy sperm and egg development.

In addition to its antioxidant properties, vitamin E also has potential benefits in improving fertility. It has been found to enhance sperm motility, which is essential for successful fertilization. Vitamin E can also improve the quality of cervical mucus, making it easier for sperm to reach the egg. This can increase the chances of conception.

Furthermore, vitamin E has been linked to improved reproductive outcomes. Studies have shown that vitamin E supplementation can increase the success rates of assisted reproductive technologies, such as in vitro fertilization (IVF). It may also reduce the risk of pregnancy complications, such as preeclampsia.

To ensure an adequate intake of vitamin E, it is recommended to include vitamin E-rich foods in your diet, such as nuts, seeds, vegetable oils, and leafy green vegetables. However, in some cases, supplementation may be necessary to meet the recommended daily intake. It is important to consult with a healthcare professional before starting any new supplement regimen.

Acetyl-L-Carnitine

Acetyl-L-Carnitine is a naturally occurring compound that plays a crucial role in both male and female fertility. This supplement has been shown to have positive effects on sperm quality, making it a potential game-changer for couples struggling with infertility.

Studies have demonstrated that acetyl-L-carnitine can improve sperm count, motility, and morphology, all of which are essential factors for successful conception. By enhancing the overall health and function of sperm, this supplement increases the chances of fertilization and pregnancy.

But acetyl-L-carnitine doesn't just benefit male fertility. It also has potential effects on female fertility, particularly in the context of assisted reproductive technologies such as in vitro fertilization (IVF) or intrauterine insemination (IUI).

Research suggests that acetyl-L-carnitine may improve the success rates of these procedures by enhancing the quality of embryos and increasing the chances of implantation. It may also help regulate hormonal balance and support overall reproductive health in women.

It's important to note that while acetyl-L-carnitine shows promise in enhancing fertility, it is always recommended to consult with a healthcare professional before adding any new supplements to your routine. They can provide personalized advice based on your specific needs and medical history.

Vitamin B12

Vitamin B12 plays a crucial role in fertility and reproductive health. A deficiency in this essential vitamin can have a significant impact on the ability to conceive and maintain a healthy pregnancy. Vitamin B12 deficiency can lead to various reproductive issues, such as irregular menstrual cycles, hormonal imbalances, and even infertility. It affects both men and women, as it is necessary for the production of healthy eggs and sperm. Supplementing with vitamin B12 can help support reproductive health by addressing any deficiencies. It can regulate menstrual cycles, promote ovulation, and improve the quality of eggs and sperm. In addition to its role in fertility, vitamin B12 is also essential for the development of a healthy baby. Adequate levels of vitamin B12 during pregnancy are crucial for proper fetal development, including the formation of the neural tube and the growth of the baby's brain and nervous system. It is important to note that vitamin B12 is primarily found in animal-based foods, such as meat, fish, dairy products, and eggs. Therefore, individuals following a vegetarian or vegan diet may be at a higher risk of vitamin B12 deficiency and may need to consider supplementation. Consulting with a healthcare professional is recommended to determine the appropriate dosage of vitamin B12 supplementation and to ensure that it is safe and suitable for individual needs. Taking vitamin B12 supplements can be a beneficial step towards supporting fertility and reproductive health.

Chasteberry

Chasteberry, also known as Vitex agnus-castus, is a natural herbal remedy that has been used for centuries to support women's reproductive health. This powerful herb has gained popularity for its potential benefits in regulating menstrual cycles, improving ovulation, and enhancing fertility.

One of the primary benefits of chasteberry is its ability to regulate hormonal imbalances that can disrupt the menstrual cycle. By acting on the pituitary gland, chasteberry helps to balance the levels of estrogen and progesterone in the body, which can result in more regular and predictable menstrual cycles.

In addition to regulating menstrual cycles, chasteberry has been found to improve ovulation in women with irregular or absent ovulation. It can stimulate the release of luteinizing hormone (LH), which is essential for triggering ovulation. By promoting regular ovulation, chasteberry can increase the chances of conception for women trying to get pregnant.

Furthermore, chasteberry has been shown to enhance fertility by improving the overall health of the reproductive system. It has anti-inflammatory properties that can reduce inflammation in the reproductive organs, creating a more favorable environment for conception. Chasteberry also supports the production of healthy cervical mucus, which is crucial for sperm survival and transport.

It is important to note that chasteberry may take time to exert its full effects on the body. It is recommended to take chasteberry supplements for at least three months to experience the maximum benefits. However, it is always advisable to consult with a healthcare professional before starting any new supplement, especially if you have any underlying medical conditions or are taking other medications.

In conclusion, chasteberry has the potential to regulate menstrual cycles, improve ovulation, and enhance fertility. By addressing hormonal imbalances and promoting a healthy reproductive system, chasteberry can be a valuable natural remedy for women trying to conceive. Consider incorporating chasteberry into your fertility journey, but always consult with a healthcare professional for personalized advice and guidance.

Magnesium

Magnesium is an essential mineral that plays a crucial role in various bodily functions, including hormone regulation and stress reduction. When it comes to fertility, magnesium has been found to have potential effects on reproductive health.

One of the main ways magnesium influences fertility is through its role in hormone regulation. Hormones play a vital role in the menstrual cycle and overall reproductive function. Magnesium helps to maintain proper hormone balance by supporting the production and activity of hormones involved in the reproductive system.

In addition to hormone regulation, magnesium also plays a role in stress reduction. Stress can have a negative impact on fertility by disrupting the delicate balance of hormones and affecting reproductive processes. Magnesium helps to calm the nervous system and reduce stress levels, which can ultimately support optimal reproductive function.

Furthermore, magnesium has potential effects on fertility due to its involvement in various biochemical reactions in the body. It is known to support energy production, DNA synthesis, and cell division, all of which are essential processes for reproductive health.

To ensure an adequate intake of magnesium, it is important to include magnesium-rich foods in your diet, such as leafy green vegetables, nuts, seeds, and whole grains. However, if you are struggling to meet your magnesium needs through diet alone, supplementation may be considered under the guidance of a healthcare professional.

In conclusion, magnesium plays a crucial role in hormone regulation, stress reduction, and potential effects on fertility. By maintaining proper hormone balance, reducing stress levels, and supporting essential biochemical reactions, magnesium can contribute to optimal reproductive health.

Selenium

Selenium is an essential mineral that plays a crucial role in both male and female fertility. It is known for its ability to support healthy sperm production and protect against oxidative stress, which can damage reproductive cells. In men, selenium is necessary for the production of healthy sperm. It helps in the formation and development of sperm cells, ensuring their proper function and motility. Adequate selenium levels have been associated with improved sperm quality and increased chances of conception. For women, selenium is important for overall reproductive health. It helps protect the eggs from oxidative damage, which can negatively impact fertility. Selenium also plays a role in the production of the thyroid hormone, which is essential for regulating the menstrual cycle and supporting healthy ovulation. Oxidative stress, caused by an imbalance between free radicals and antioxidants in the body, can have detrimental effects on fertility. Selenium acts as a powerful antioxidant, neutralizing harmful free radicals and reducing oxidative stress. By protecting reproductive cells from damage, selenium can enhance fertility and increase the chances of successful conception. It is important to note that selenium levels should be balanced, as both deficiency and excess can have adverse effects on fertility. While selenium is necessary for reproductive health, excessive intake can be harmful. Therefore, it is recommended to consult with a healthcare professional to determine the appropriate selenium supplementation for optimal fertility.

Evening Primrose Oil

Evening primrose oil is a natural supplement that has gained attention for its potential benefits in supporting cervical mucus production, hormone balance, and fertility.

Derived from the seeds of the evening primrose plant, this oil is rich in gamma-linolenic acid (GLA), an omega-6 fatty acid with anti-inflammatory properties.

One of the key benefits of evening primrose oil is its ability to support cervical mucus production. Cervical mucus plays a crucial role in fertility as it helps sperm travel through the reproductive tract and reach the egg. Insufficient or poor-quality cervical mucus can hinder conception. Evening primrose oil has been found to improve the quality and quantity of cervical mucus, creating a more favorable environment for sperm.

In addition to supporting cervical mucus production, evening primrose oil may also help balance hormones. Hormonal imbalances can disrupt the menstrual cycle and negatively impact fertility. GLA in evening primrose oil has been shown to regulate hormone levels and reduce symptoms associated with hormonal fluctuations, such as mood swings and breast tenderness.

Furthermore, evening primrose oil has been studied for its potential role in enhancing fertility. Some research suggests that the GLA content in evening primrose oil may improve the overall reproductive health of women, increasing the chances of successful conception. However, further studies are needed to fully understand the extent of its fertility-enhancing effects.

It is important to note that evening primrose oil should be used under the guidance of a healthcare professional, especially for individuals with underlying medical conditions or those taking medications. As with any supplement, it is crucial to consult with a healthcare provider before incorporating evening primrose oil into your fertility regimen.

Green Tea Extract

Green tea extract is derived from the leaves of the Camellia sinensis plant and is known for its antioxidant properties. Antioxidants help protect the body from oxidative damage caused by free radicals, which can contribute to various health issues, including infertility.

Research suggests that green tea extract may have potential benefits for reproductive health and fertility. The antioxidants found in green tea extract, such as catechins and polyphenols, have been shown to have positive effects on sperm quality and function. They can help reduce oxidative stress and improve sperm motility, which are essential factors for successful conception.

In addition to its effects on male fertility, green tea extract may also have potential benefits for female reproductive health. It has been found to support hormonal balance, which is crucial for regular menstrual cycles and ovulation. Green tea extract may also help reduce inflammation in the reproductive system, creating a more favorable environment for conception.

It is important to note that while green tea extract may offer potential benefits for fertility, it should be consumed in moderation. Excessive consumption of green tea or green tea extract may have negative effects on fertility due to its caffeine content. High levels of caffeine intake have been associated with decreased fertility and an increased risk of miscarriage.

If you are considering incorporating green tea extract into your fertility regimen, it is advisable to consult with a healthcare professional or fertility specialist. They can provide personalized guidance based on your specific needs and circumstances.

L-Arginine

L-Arginine plays a crucial role in improving blood flow to the reproductive organs, making it a valuable supplement for enhancing fertility. This essential amino acid is converted into nitric oxide in the body, which helps to relax and dilate blood vessels, promoting better circulation. By increasing blood flow to the reproductive organs, L-arginine can improve the delivery of oxygen and nutrients, supporting their optimal function.

In addition to its role in improving blood flow, L-arginine also offers potential benefits for fertility. Studies have shown that this amino acid can enhance sperm production and quality in men. It may help to increase sperm count, improve motility, and enhance overall sperm health. For women, L-arginine can promote a healthy uterine lining and support proper implantation of a fertilized egg.

Supplementing with L-arginine can be particularly beneficial for couples who are struggling with infertility due to poor blood circulation or reproductive issues. By improving blood flow to the reproductive organs, L-arginine may increase the chances of successful conception and pregnancy. However, it is important to note that individual results may vary, and it is always advisable to consult with a healthcare professional before starting any new supplementation regimen.

Maca Root

Maca Root:

Maca root is a natural supplement that has been used for centuries as a fertility enhancer. It is derived from the root of the maca plant, which is native to the Andes Mountains of Peru. This powerful herb is known for its ability to balance hormones, boost libido, and improve fertility.

One of the key benefits of maca root is its effect on hormone balance. It contains unique compounds called macaenes and macamides, which have been shown to regulate hormonal production in the body. This can be particularly beneficial for women who are experiencing hormonal imbalances that may be affecting their fertility.

Additionally, maca root has been found to increase libido in both men and women. It is believed to work by stimulating the production of sex hormones, such as testosterone and estrogen, which can enhance sexual desire and improve overall reproductive health.

Furthermore, maca root has been traditionally used as a fertility enhancer. It is believed to support healthy egg development and improve the quality of sperm, increasing the chances of successful conception. The nutrients found in maca root, including vitamins, minerals, and antioxidants, nourish the reproductive system and promote optimal fertility.

Incorporating maca root into your daily routine can be done through supplementation or by adding the powdered form to smoothies, baked goods, or other recipes. It is generally considered safe for most people, but it's always a good idea to consult with a healthcare professional before starting any new supplement.

In conclusion, maca root is a natural supplement that offers a range of benefits for hormone balance, libido, and fertility. Its traditional use as a fertility enhancer has been supported by scientific research, making it a popular choice for couples trying to conceive. Consider adding maca root to your fertility regimen to support your reproductive health and increase your chances of achieving pregnancy.

Vitamin A

Vitamin A plays a crucial role in reproductive health, as it is essential for both fetal development and sperm production. This powerful vitamin is involved in the growth and differentiation of cells, making it vital for the development of the reproductive organs in both males and females.

During pregnancy, vitamin A is particularly important for the healthy development of the fetus. It is involved in the formation of the eyes, lungs, heart, and other vital organs. Adequate intake of vitamin A can help prevent birth defects and ensure the proper growth and development of the baby.

For men, vitamin A is essential for sperm production. It helps in the production of healthy sperm and plays a role in maintaining the integrity of the sperm DNA. A deficiency in vitamin A can lead to decreased sperm count and motility, which can impact fertility.

In addition to its role in reproductive health, vitamin A also supports the immune system, promotes healthy skin and vision, and plays a role in bone growth and maintenance. It is found in a variety of foods, including liver, eggs, dairy products, and colorful fruits and vegetables.

To ensure adequate intake of vitamin A, it is important to maintain a balanced diet that includes a variety of vitamin A-rich foods. However, it is important to note that excessive intake of vitamin A can be harmful, especially during pregnancy. Therefore, it is recommended to consult with a healthcare professional to determine the appropriate intake of vitamin A for your specific needs.

Choline

Choline is an essential nutrient that plays a crucial role in fertility and reproductive health. It is particularly important for healthy egg development and neural tube formation. Choline is a water-soluble vitamin-like compound that is found in foods such as eggs, liver, and fish.

One of the main functions of choline in fertility is its involvement in the production of phospholipids, which are vital for the formation of cell membranes. This is especially important during the early stages of pregnancy when rapid cell division and growth occur. Adequate choline intake can help ensure the healthy development of the neural tube, which eventually becomes the brain and spinal cord of the fetus.

In addition to its role in neural tube formation, choline also helps support healthy egg development. It is involved in the production of acetylcholine, a neurotransmitter that plays a role in regulating ovarian function. Adequate choline levels can help optimize egg quality and increase the chances of successful fertilization.

Furthermore, choline has been found to have antioxidant properties, which can help protect reproductive cells from oxidative damage. This is particularly important for both male and female fertility, as oxidative stress can negatively impact sperm and egg quality. By reducing oxidative stress, choline may improve overall reproductive health and increase the chances of conception.

It is important to note that choline requirements can vary depending on factors such as age, sex, and life stage. Pregnant women, in particular, have higher choline needs to support the developing fetus. However, many individuals do not meet their recommended choline intake through diet alone. In such cases, choline supplements can be beneficial in ensuring adequate levels of this important nutrient.

In conclusion, choline plays a vital role in fertility and reproductive health. It supports healthy egg development and neural tube formation, and may also have antioxidant properties that protect reproductive cells. Meeting the recommended choline intake through diet or supplementation can help optimize fertility and increase the chances of a successful pregnancy.

Black Cohosh

Black cohosh, also known as Actaea racemosa, is a herbal supplement that has been used for centuries to support women's reproductive health. It is commonly used to regulate menstrual cycles, reduce menopausal symptoms, and even support fertility.

One of the primary benefits of black cohosh is its ability to regulate menstrual cycles. Many women experience irregular periods, which can make it difficult to track ovulation and increase the chances of conception. Black cohosh helps to balance hormone levels in the body, which can lead to more regular and predictable menstrual cycles.

In addition to regulating menstrual cycles, black cohosh has also been found to be effective in reducing menopausal symptoms. Menopause is a natural transition that every woman goes through, but it can be accompanied by uncomfortable symptoms such as hot flashes, night sweats, and mood swings. Black cohosh has been shown to alleviate these symptoms and improve overall quality of life during this stage of life.

Furthermore, black cohosh has shown potential in supporting fertility. It helps to balance hormone levels, which is crucial for healthy ovulation and the development of a receptive uterine lining. By promoting hormonal balance, black cohosh may increase the chances of successful conception and pregnancy.

It is important to note that while black cohosh has been used for centuries and has shown promising results, it is always recommended to consult with a healthcare professional before starting any new supplement. They can provide personalized guidance and ensure that black cohosh is safe and appropriate for individual needs.

Garlic

Garlic, a popular ingredient in various cuisines, not only adds flavor to dishes but also offers potential benefits for reproductive health. Research suggests that garlic may have positive effects on sperm quality, hormone balance, and overall reproductive health.

When it comes to sperm quality, garlic has been found to have antioxidant properties that can help protect sperm cells from oxidative damage. Oxidative stress can negatively impact sperm health, leading to reduced sperm count, motility, and morphology. By reducing oxidative stress, garlic may contribute to improved sperm quality and fertility.

In addition to its potential effects on sperm quality, garlic may also play a role in hormone balance. Hormonal imbalances can disrupt the menstrual cycle in women and affect sperm production in men. Garlic contains compounds that have been shown to regulate hormone levels, potentially helping to restore balance and improve reproductive health.

Furthermore, garlic has been associated with various health benefits, including cardiovascular health and immune system support. A healthy cardiovascular system is essential for optimal reproductive function, as it ensures proper blood flow to the reproductive organs. Garlic's ability to improve blood circulation may indirectly benefit fertility by enhancing the delivery of nutrients and oxygen to the reproductive system.

It's important to note that while garlic shows promise in supporting reproductive health, further research is needed to fully understand its mechanisms and potential benefits. As with any supplement, it's always advisable to consult with a healthcare professional before incorporating garlic or any other supplement into your fertility regimen.

Vitamin K

Vitamin K plays a crucial role in fertility, with its impact extending to blood clotting, bone health, and fetal development. This essential vitamin is involved in the production of clotting factors, which are necessary for proper blood clotting. During pregnancy, vitamin K ensures the formation of a healthy placenta and helps prevent excessive bleeding during childbirth.

In addition to its role in blood clotting, vitamin K also contributes to bone health. It helps activate proteins that are responsible for binding calcium to the bone matrix, promoting bone mineralization and strength. Adequate vitamin K levels are especially important during pregnancy, as the growing fetus relies on the mother's calcium stores for bone development.

Furthermore, vitamin K plays a vital role in fetal development. It is involved in the synthesis of certain proteins that are essential for normal growth and development. These proteins contribute to the formation of the nervous system, including the brain and spinal cord.

To ensure sufficient vitamin K intake, it is recommended to include foods rich in this vitamin in your diet. Green leafy vegetables, such as kale and spinach, are excellent sources of vitamin K. Other sources include broccoli, Brussels sprouts, and fermented foods like sauerkraut. Supplementation may be necessary for individuals with specific dietary restrictions or those who have difficulty meeting their vitamin K needs through food alone.

Resveratrol

Resveratrol is a natural compound found in various plants, including grapes, berries, and peanuts. It has gained attention for its antioxidant properties and potential benefits for reproductive health and fertility. Antioxidants are substances that help protect cells from damage caused by free radicals, unstable molecules that can harm the body's cells and DNA.

Research suggests that resveratrol may have positive effects on reproductive health by reducing oxidative stress and inflammation. Oxidative stress occurs when there is an imbalance between free radicals and the body's antioxidant defenses. This imbalance can lead to cellular damage and has been linked to infertility and reproductive disorders.

Studies have shown that resveratrol may help improve sperm quality and motility in men. It may also support female reproductive health by promoting healthy egg development and reducing oxidative damage to the ovaries. Additionally, resveratrol has been found to have anti-inflammatory effects, which may further contribute to its potential benefits for fertility.

While more research is needed to fully understand the effects of resveratrol on reproductive health and fertility, its antioxidant properties make it a promising supplement for those trying to conceive. It is important to note that supplements should be used in consultation with a healthcare professional, as individual needs and circumstances may vary.

Nettle Leaf

Nettle leaf, also known as stinging nettle, is a powerful herb that offers numerous potential benefits for hormonal balance, inflammation reduction, and fertility improvement. This natural remedy has been used for centuries in traditional medicine to support overall health and well-being.

One of the key advantages of nettle leaf is its ability to support hormonal balance. Hormonal imbalances can disrupt the menstrual cycle and affect fertility. Nettle leaf contains compounds that help regulate hormone levels, promoting a healthy balance and improving reproductive function.

In addition to hormonal balance, nettle leaf also possesses anti-inflammatory properties. Inflammation in the reproductive organs can hinder conception and affect fertility. By reducing inflammation, nettle leaf creates a more favorable environment for conception and supports overall reproductive health.

Moreover, nettle leaf has been found to have positive effects on fertility. It is believed to improve sperm quality and motility in men, increasing the chances of successful fertilization. For women, nettle leaf can help in the regulation of menstrual cycles, promoting regular ovulation and enhancing the chances of conception.

To incorporate nettle leaf into your fertility-enhancing routine, you can consume it in various forms. Nettle leaf tea is a popular option and can be easily prepared by steeping dried nettle leaves in hot water. You can also find nettle leaf supplements in capsule or tincture form, which provide a concentrated dose of its beneficial compounds.

As with any herbal remedy, it is important to consult with a healthcare professional before incorporating nettle leaf into your fertility regimen, especially if you have any underlying health conditions or are taking medications. They can provide guidance on the appropriate dosage and ensure it is safe for you to use.

In conclusion, nettle leaf offers potential benefits for supporting hormonal balance, reducing inflammation, and improving fertility. By incorporating this natural remedy into your routine, you may enhance your chances of conception and promote overall reproductive health.

Antioxidant Blend

An antioxidant blend is a combination of various antioxidants that work together to protect reproductive cells from oxidative damage and improve fertility outcomes.

Oxidative stress, caused by an imbalance between free radicals and antioxidants in the body, can negatively impact fertility by damaging sperm, eggs, and reproductive organs.

Antioxidants are substances that help neutralize free radicals and prevent oxidative damage. They play a crucial role in maintaining reproductive health and increasing the chances of conception. An antioxidant blend provides a synergistic effect, as different antioxidants work together to enhance their individual benefits.

By taking an antioxidant blend, individuals can support their reproductive system by reducing oxidative stress and improving overall fertility. These blends typically contain a combination of vitamins, minerals, and plant-based antioxidants, such as vitamins C and E, selenium, zinc, and coenzyme Q10.

Research has shown that antioxidant blends can have several positive effects on fertility outcomes. They can improve sperm quality and motility, enhance egg quality and maturation, and support healthy hormone balance. Additionally, antioxidant blends have been found to reduce inflammation in the reproductive system, which can further enhance fertility.

It's important to note that while antioxidant blends can be beneficial for fertility, they should be taken as part of a comprehensive approach to reproductive health. This includes maintaining a balanced diet, exercising regularly, managing stress, and avoiding harmful substances.

In conclusion, antioxidant blends offer a range of benefits for protecting reproductive cells from oxidative damage and improving fertility outcomes. By incorporating these blends into their daily routine, individuals can support their reproductive health and increase their chances of conceiving.

Ashwagandha

Ashwagandha, also known as Withania somnifera, is an ancient herb that has been used in traditional Ayurvedic medicine for centuries. It is known for its adaptogenic properties, meaning it helps the body adapt to stress and promotes overall well-being. But what does ashwagandha have to do with fertility?

Research suggests that ashwagandha may play a role in enhancing fertility by reducing stress levels and balancing hormones. Stress can have a negative impact on reproductive health, as it can disrupt the delicate balance of hormones needed for ovulation and sperm production. By reducing stress, ashwagandha may help restore hormonal balance and improve fertility.

In addition to its stress-reducing properties, ashwagandha has also been shown to have potential benefits for male fertility. Studies have found that ashwagandha supplementation can improve sperm quality, including sperm count, motility, and morphology. This may increase the chances of successful conception for couples trying to conceive.

Furthermore, ashwagandha has been found to have antioxidant properties, which can help protect reproductive cells from oxidative damage. Oxidative stress can negatively impact fertility by causing damage to sperm and eggs. By reducing oxidative stress, ashwagandha may improve reproductive health and increase the chances of successful pregnancy.

It is important to note that while ashwagandha shows promise in enhancing fertility, more research is needed to fully understand its effects and optimal dosage. As with any supplement, it is always recommended to consult with a healthcare professional before starting ashwagandha or any other fertility-enhancing supplement.

Chromium

Chromium:

Chromium is an essential mineral that plays a crucial role in glucose metabolism. It is involved in the regulation of insulin, a hormone that helps control blood sugar levels. Proper glucose metabolism is not only important for overall health but also for fertility and reproductive health.

When it comes to fertility, maintaining stable blood sugar levels is crucial. Fluctuations in blood sugar can negatively impact reproductive hormones and disrupt the menstrual cycle. Chromium helps improve insulin sensitivity and promote more stable blood sugar levels, which in turn can support reproductive health.

Research suggests that chromium supplementation may have potential benefits for fertility. It may help regulate menstrual cycles and improve ovulation, increasing the chances of conception. Additionally, stable blood sugar levels can reduce the risk of conditions such as polycystic ovary syndrome (PCOS), which can affect fertility.

Furthermore, chromium's role in glucose metabolism can also have positive effects on male fertility. Studies have shown that chromium supplementation may improve sperm quality and motility, enhancing the chances of successful fertilization.

Incorporating chromium-rich foods into your diet or considering chromium supplementation can be beneficial for fertility and reproductive health. However, it is important to consult with a healthcare professional before starting any new supplements to ensure they are appropriate for your individual needs.

Frequently Asked Questions

- **What is the role of folic acid in fertility?**

  Folic acid plays a crucial role in preventing birth defects and supporting healthy ovulation and sperm production. It is essential for the proper development of the neural tube in the early stages of pregnancy. Supplementing with folic acid before conception and during early pregnancy can significantly reduce the risk of neural tube defects.

- **Why is iron important for fertility?**

  Iron deficiency can negatively impact fertility in both men and women. In women, iron deficiency anemia can lead to irregular menstrual cycles and decreased egg quality. In men, iron deficiency can affect sperm production and motility. Supplementing with iron can help improve fertility outcomes for couples trying to conceive.

- **How does vitamin D deficiency affect fertility?**

  Vitamin D deficiency has been linked to decreased fertility in both men and women. It plays a crucial role in reproductive health, including hormone regulation and egg development. Supplementing with vitamin D can help improve fertility by addressing any deficiencies and supporting optimal reproductive function.

- **What is the role of Coenzyme Q10 in fertility?**

  Coenzyme Q10 (CoQ10) is known for its antioxidant properties and its potential benefits in enhancing egg quality and sperm motility. It helps protect reproductive cells from oxidative damage and supports overall reproductive health. Supplementing with CoQ10 may be beneficial for couples trying to conceive.

- **How does vitamin C affect fertility?**

  Vitamin C is a powerful antioxidant that can positively impact sperm quality and female reproductive health. It helps protect reproductive cells from oxidative stress and supports the overall functioning of the reproductive system. Including vitamin C-rich foods in your diet or taking a supplement may be beneficial for fertility.

- **Why is zinc important for fertility?**

Zinc plays a crucial role in fertility as it is involved in hormone regulation and sperm production. It is essential for both male and female reproductive health. Supplementing with zinc can help optimize fertility by addressing any deficiencies and supporting proper reproductive function.

- **What are the benefits of omega-3 fatty acids for fertility?**

Omega-3 fatty acids have been shown to improve fertility by reducing inflammation and supporting reproductive health. They can help regulate hormone levels, improve egg quality, and enhance sperm function. Including omega-3-rich foods in your diet or taking a supplement may be beneficial for fertility.

- **How does gut health affect fertility?**

Gut health plays a significant role in fertility as it impacts nutrient absorption, hormone regulation, and immune function. Probiotics, which are beneficial bacteria, can help support a healthy gut microbiome and improve fertility outcomes for both men and women. Supplementing with probiotics may be beneficial for fertility.

- **What is the role of calcium in reproductive health?**

Calcium is essential for proper hormone function and egg fertilization. It plays a crucial role in the overall reproductive health of both men and women. Ensuring an adequate intake of calcium through diet or supplementation can help support fertility and reproductive function.

- **How does vitamin E affect fertility?**

Vitamin E is an antioxidant that helps protect reproductive cells from oxidative damage. It may have potential benefits in improving fertility and reproductive outcomes. Including vitamin E-rich foods in your diet or taking a supplement may be beneficial for fertility.

Have Questions / Comments?

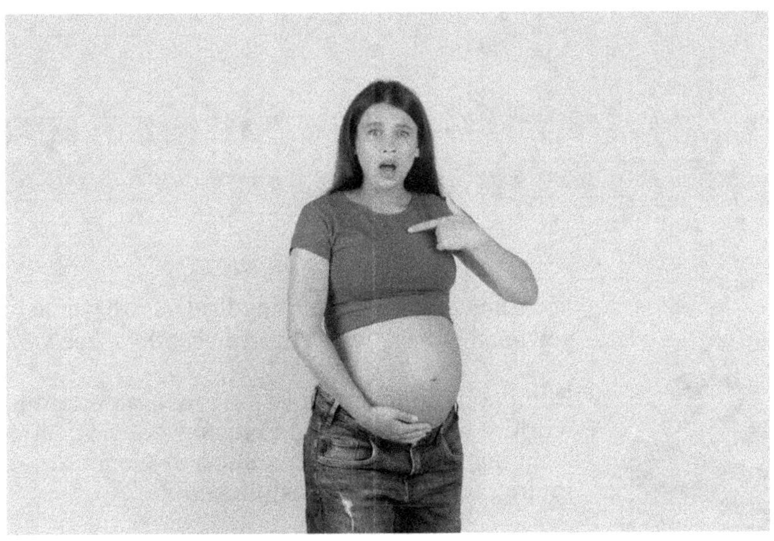

This book was designed to cover as much info as possible but I know I have probably missed something, or some new amazing discovery that has just come out.

If you notice something missing or have a question that I failed to answer, please get in touch and let me know. If I can, I will email you an answer and also update the book so others can also benefit from it.

Thanks For Being Awesome :)

Submit Your Questions / Comments At:
<u>Get In Touch Babydreamers.net</u>

Get How To Be A Super Mom 100% FREE

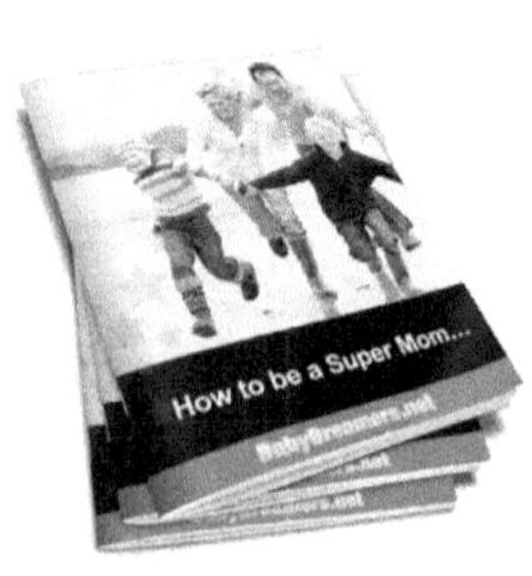

For being one of our amazing readers, we would love to offer you another book we have created, 100% free.

Being a mom is probably the most important job in the world – we've all heard that, and it's true. You're bringing up the next generation of wonderful, intelligent, loving, creative, responsible people.

We all want to be Super Mom and to be everything and do everything, but it this possible?

Being a Super Mom is possible, but you have to learn how to empower yourself to be the kind of Super Mom that you feel you need to be, keeping in mind that the title Super Mom doesn't mean the same thing to everyone.

Get How to be a Super Mom For Free

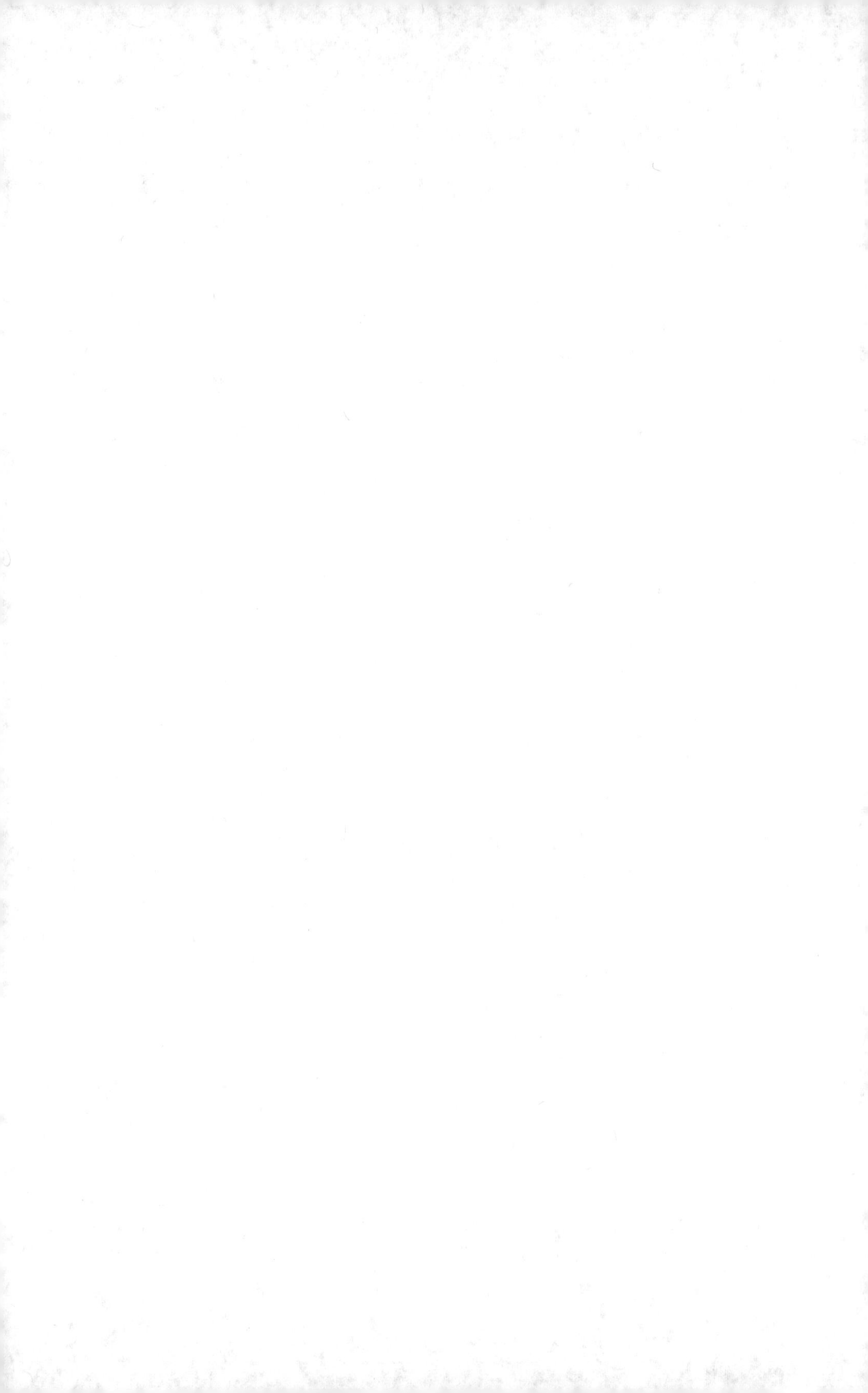